THE 30 DAY'S DASH DIET MEAL PLAN

Recipes and Life Hacks to Maintain Low Sodium Levels by Eating Different

Fit Chef Dash

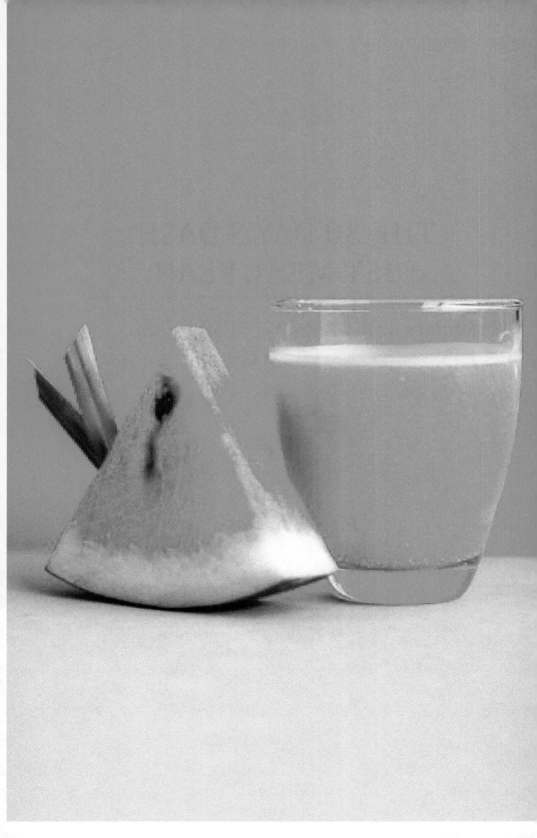

Table of Contents

INTRODUCTION

The Dash diet is a dietary approach to treat hypertension. It helps to maintain, improve, and support overall health as well as lowering blood pressure. The diet was created by the National Institute of Health as a way to treat hypertension without medication. The main idea of the Dash diet is to reduce the amount of sodium in food while eating nutrients that help to maintain normal blood pressure. These nutrients are calcium, potassium, and magnesium.

The Dash diet can give you awesome results in just two weeks. The nutrition plan is a scientifically proved system designed by physicians to reduce your blood pressure up to 15.

It also helps with weight loss and in preventing heart disease, cancer, osteoporosis, diabetes, and stroke. It is not a restrictive diet; it is a lifestyle that can be followed with very little adjustment. If your goal is weight loss, the Dash diet can be personalized by a nutritionist or doctor because its standard form wasn't designed for that purpose.

Dash Diet for Weight Loss and to Lower Blood Pressure

For the last few years, the Dash diet has been one of the highest rated of the most popular diets. It has proven to be effective in fighting high blood pressure.

According to the National Institutes of Health, the success of the diet in weight loss is 3.3 points out of 5 and 4.8 points out of 5 in neutralizing and lowering blood pressure. The major cause of high blood pressure is dietary sodium. Excessive concentration of sodium leads to deposits in the blood vessels walls. The chemical composition of sodium attracts water, which causes swelling and narrowing of the blood vessels. Therefore, the blood pressure rises and causes hypertension.

Studies suggested that on average during a 70-yearlifespan, a person can eat approximately half a ton of salt. This is the only mineral that we eat in its pure form. It doesn't mean that salt is harmful to our bodies. Like every mineral, it has benefits and is imperative for regulating the water-salt balance in the body, the formation of gastric juice, and the transfer of oxygen in blood cells. However, when it is present in excessive amounts, it can be a disaster.

The Dash diet allows you to decrease the amount of sodium in your body. The recommended daily amount of sodium should not exceed 2300mg. Some studies show that reducing the amount of sodium to 1500mg can help to control high blood pressure.

The diet is balanced with nutrients that are very important for normal blood pressure such as potassium, magnesium, calcium, protein, and plant fibers. The perfect combination of these nutrients will give remarkable results.

The Dash diet is the perfect combination of different food groups such as fruits, vegetables, grains, dairy products, meat, fish, poultry, eggs, nuts and seeds, legumes, and oils. In addition, you will consume less salt, sugar, and fatty foods, which are a cause of high blood cholesterol. If you follow the diet strictly and do physical activity every day, it is possible to lose 17-19 lbsin4 months.

The major advantage of dash eating is that it is based on the body's natural eating patterns. And the lost weight doesn't return if you adopt it as a lifestyle. The dash diet is considered one of the healthiest diets. Although it was created for hypertensive patients, it can improve the well-being and health of anyone.

What to Eat and Avoid on Dash Diet:

Grains

In this diet, you can have whole-grains, which are rich in fiber and nutrients. It is easy to find low-fat versions to substitute for the high-fat choices.

What to Eat	Eat Occasionally	What to avoid
Whole grain breakfast cereals	Whole wheat noodles and pasta	White bread
Bulgur		Regular pasta
Popcorn		White rice
Rice cakes		
Brown rice		
Quinoa		

Fresh Vegetables

Vegetables are the richest source of fiber, vitamins, potassium, and magnesium. You can have them whenever and in whatever quantity you want.

What to Eat	What to avoid
All seasonal and fresh vegetables Low sodium canned vegetables	Regular canned vegetables

Fruits and Berries

The fruits and berries have the same imperative benefits as vegetables. They are rich in minerals and vitamins. The fruits and berries are low-fat content. They are a good replacement for desserts and snacks. Fruit peels have the highest amount of fiber and nutrients in comparison with fruit flesh.

What to Eat	Eat Occasionally	What to Avoid
All fresh fruits and berries such as apple, pineapple, strawberries, etc	Citrus fruits	Canned fruits Coconut

Dairy

Dairy products are the main source of vitamin D and calcium. The only limit for the dash diet is saturated and high-fat dairy food. You can replace dairy products with nut, almond, cashew, and soy milk.

What to Eat	Eat Occasionally	What to Avoid
Low-fat or fat-free cheese	Low-fat cream	Full-fat cream
Low-fat or fat-free yogurt	Low-fat buttermilk	Full-fat milk
Low-fat or fat-free milk		Full-fat cheese
Low-fat or fat-free skim milk		Full-fat yogurt
Low-fat or fat-free frozen yogurt		

Meat and Poultry

Meat is rich in B vitamins, protein, zinc, and iron. You can have meat in all different styles and varieties. You can broil, grill, bake, or roast it. Make sure not to eat skin and fat from poultry and meat.

What to Eat	Eat Occasionally	What to Avoid
Skinless chicken	Lean cuts of red meat (pork, beef, veal, lamb)	Fat cuts of meat
Chicken fillet	Eggs	Pork belly
		Bacon
		Fat

Fish and Seafood

Fish, which is high in omega-3 fatty acids, is beneficial. All types of seafood and fish are allowed on the dash diet, but choose wisely with high omega-3.

What to Eat	What to avoid
Salmon	High sodium canned fish and seafood
Herring	

Nuts, Seeds, and Legumes

Nuts, seeds, and legumes are rich in fiber, phyto chemicals, potassium, magnesium, and proteins. They help to fight cancer and cardiovascular disease. They are high in calories and should be eaten in moderation.

What to Eat
All types of seeds
All types of nuts
All types of legumes

Fats and Oils

The main function of dietary fat is to help in absorbing vitamins. High amounts of fat can lead to increased heart disease, obesity, and diabetes.
According to the dash diet, your daily meal plan shouldn't include more than 30 percent of daily calories from fat.

What to Eat	Eat Occasionally	What to Avoid
Margarine	Low-fat	Butter
Vegetable	mayonnaise	Lard
oils	Light salad	Solid
	dressings	shortening

Sweets

You don't have to cut sweets out of your daily diet but there are some restrictions in the Dash diet.

- Choose sugar-free, low-fat/fat-free sweets
- Replace dessert with fruits and berries

What to Eat	Eat Occasionally	What to Avoid
Fruit/berries	Hard candy	Biscuits
sorbets	Aspartame (NutraSweet,	Crackers
Fruit ice	Equal)	Cookies
Graham crackers	Agave syrup	Soda
Honey	Maple syrup	Unrefined
Sugar-free fruit		sugar
jelly		Table sugar
		Sweet junk
		food

Alcohol and Caffeine

Limit alcohol to two drinks per day for men and one for women. Alcohol and caffeine intake may be restricted by a doctor.

Best Tips for the Dash Diet

- **Physical activity and walking is vital**

  Exercising and walking will enhance the effect of the Dash diet and will help in weight loss too. To stabilize the blood pressure, the perfect combo is a minimum of two hours of walking and 30minutesof exercise per week.

- **Avoid drastic life changes**

  Avoid stressing your body by suddenly changing your eating habits. Go step-by-step until your body adjusts to the new diet.

- **Keep a food journal**

  Keeping a food journal will help you control your food intake and make significant changes in your attitude to food.

- **Make green your compulsory meal partner**

  Make a rule to add green vegetables to every meal. This will provide fiber and potassium.

- **Become a vegetarian**

  Limiting your meat consumption is a very healthy option. Start eating meat no more than once per week. Instead, eat beans, nuts, tofu, and other protein-rich foods.

- **Fresh box in your kitchen**

  Make a fresh box with fruits, vegetables, and rice cakes for snacks. This will help you to resist the temptation of high-sodium junk food.

- **Reading food labels is useful**

  Always read the nutrition labels before buying processed food. Keep in mind that low-sodium canned food must have less than 140mg of sodium per serving.

- **Add spices to life**

  Spices such as rosemary, cayenne pepper, chili pepper, cilantro, dill, cinnamon, etc. can enhance the flavor and appeal of your low-salt meals.

- **Give yourself good snack choices**

  Different types of snacks appeal to different people. It can be a difficult step to switch completely to healthy food. That's why it helps to make a list of your favorite snacks. The food list will change as you get rid of all junk food from your diet.

- **Get a physical examination every two months**

  Some health problems can't be changed by diet alone. Getting a doctor's advice is important. Go in for a physical before starting a diet and then consult a doctor every two months to keep yourself on track and maintain control of your health.

BREAKFAST

Baked French Toasts

8 Serving

Preparation time: 18 minutes

Ingredients:

- 8-12 drops liquid stevia
- 4 tbsps olive oil
- 8 eggs
- 8 (¾-inch thick) white bread slices, trimmed and sliced diagonally
- 10 cups unsweetened almond milk

Directions:

- Preheat the oven to 400 °F. Arrange a baking sheet in the oven to heat. In a bowl, add almond milk and eggs and beat slightly.
- Dip each bread slice in an egg mixture evenly. In a skillet, heat oil over medium heat. Add bread slices, one at a time, and cook for about 1 minute per side.
- Now, arrange the slices onto hot baking sheet in a single layer—Bake for about 4 minutes.
- Serve warm.

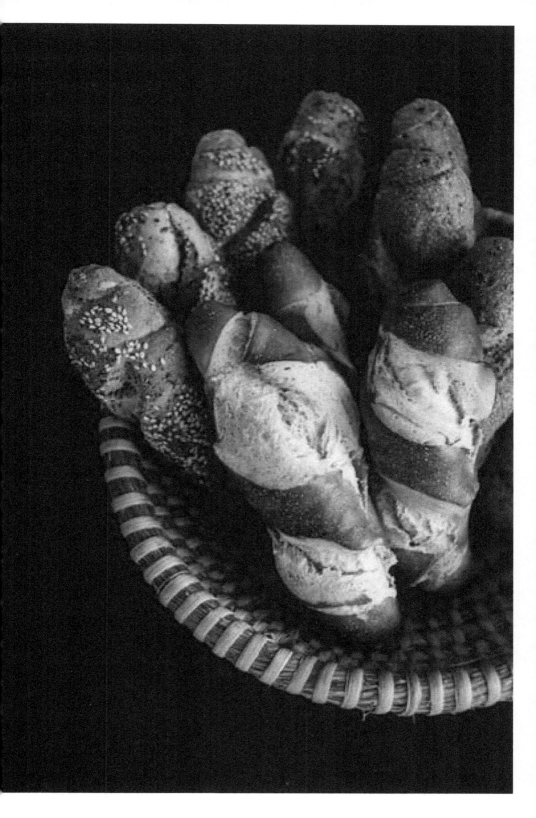

Microwave Egg Scramble

4 Serving

Preparation time: 10 minutes and 1½ minutes

Ingredients:
- 8 egg whites
- Freshly ground black pepper, to taste
- 4 eggs
- 0.5cup fresh mushrooms, chopped finely
- 0.5 CUP fat-free milk

Directions:
- Grease 2 (12-oz.) coffee mugs. In a bowl, add milk, eggs, and egg whites and beat until well combined. Stir in mushrooms. Divide the egg mixture into prepared mugs evenly and microwave on High for about 45 seconds. Remove the mugs from the microwave and stir well. Microwave for about 30-45 seconds more. Serve immediately.

Cheesy Scrambled Eggs

12 Serving

Preparation time: 18 minutes

Ingredients:
- 4 tbsps fresh chives, chopped finely
- 4 tbsps unsalted margarine
- 2 small red onion, chopped
- Pinch of salt
- 2 jalapeño pepper, seeded and chopped
- 24 eggs, beaten lightly
- Freshly ground black pepper, to taste
- 8 oz. goat cheese, crumbled

Directions:
- In a large skillet, melt margarine over medium heat and sauté the jalapeño pepper and onion for about 4-5 minutes. Add eggs, salt, and black pepper and cook for about 3 minutes, stirring continuously.
- Remove from heat and immediately stir in chives and cheese.
- Serve immediately.

Apple Omelet

4 Serving

Preparation time: 20 minutes

Ingredients:

- 2 tsps unsweetened applesauce
- 2 large green apple, cored and sliced thinly
- 8 eggs
- Pinch of salt
- 6 tsps olive oil, divided
- 0.5 tsp. ground cinnamon
- 0.25 tsp. organic vanilla extract

Directions:

- **In** a non-stick frying pan, heat 1 tsp. of oil over medium-low heat. Add apple slices and sprinkle with cinnamon and nutmeg. Cook for about 4-5 minutes, turning once halfway through. Meanwhile, in a bowl, add eggs, vanilla extract, and salt and beat until fluffy. Add remaining oil in the pan and let it heat completely. Place the egg mixture over apple slices evenly and cook for about 3-4 minutes or until desired doneness. Carefully turn the pan over a serving plate and immediately fold the omelet. Serve with the drizzling of applesauce.

Spinach Omelet

4 Serving

Preparation time: 25 minutes

Ingredients:

- 1 cup water
- 1 cuptomato, seeded and chopped finely
- 4 tbsps. olive oil
- 1 tsp. cumin seeds
- Freshly ground black pepper, to taste
- 10 cups fresh spinach, chopped finely
- 2 small green chili, seeded and chopped finely
- 1.5 cups chickpea flour
- Pinch of salt

Directions:

- In a bowl, mix together cumin seeds, salt, and black pepper.
- Slowly add the water and mix until a smooth mixture forms. Add spinach, tomato, and green chili and mix until well combined.
- In a non-stick skillet, heat 1 tbsp. of oil over medium heat. Add the spinach mixture and tilt the pan to spread it.

- Cook for about 5-7 minutes. Place remaining oil over the omelet and carefully flip the side. Cook for about 4-5 minutes or until golden brown.

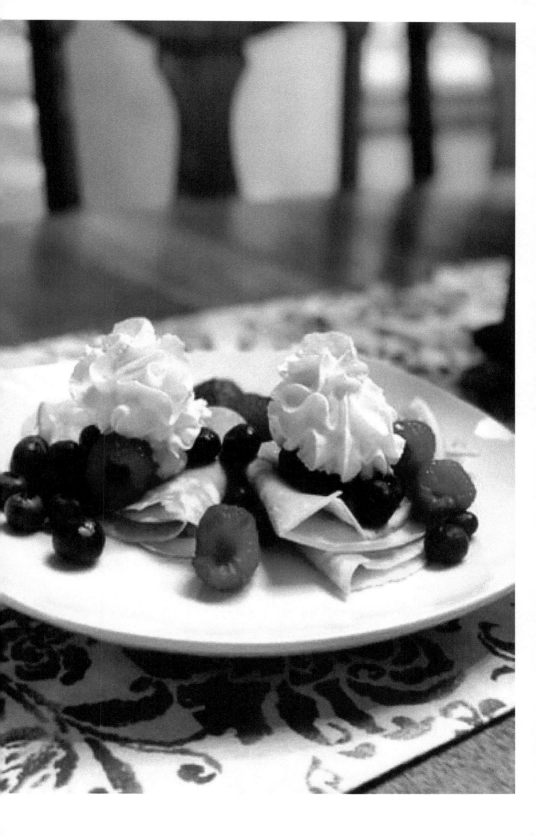

8 Serving

Preparation time: 32 minutes

Ingredients:

- 6-8 tbsps of water
- Pinch of salt
- 6 tbsp. feta cheese, crumbled
- 14 cups fresh baby spinach
- 8eggs
- Freshly ground black pepper, to taste

Directions:

- Preheat the oven to 400 °F. Lightly grease 2 small baking dishes.
- In a large frying pan, add spinach and water over medium heat and cook for about 3-4 minutes.
- Remove from heat and drain the excess water completely.
- Divide the spinach into prepared baking dishes evenly.
- Carefully crack 2 eggs in each baking dish over spinach.
- Sprinkle with salt and black pepper and top with feta cheese evenly.

- Arrange the baking dishes onto a large cookie sheet.
- Bake for about 15-18 minutes.
- Remove from oven and set aside for about 5 minutes before serving.

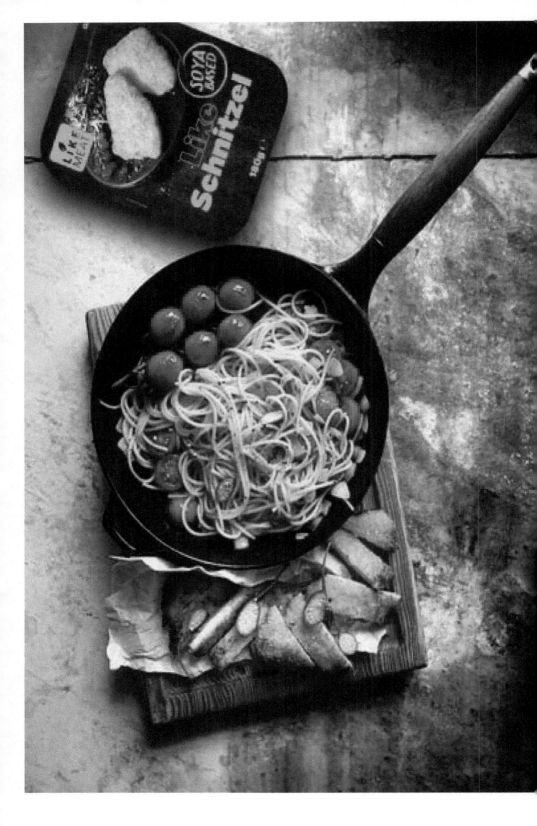

Spaghetti Frittata

5 Servings

Preparation time: 20 minutes
Ingredients:

- 4 tsps olive oil
- 4 oz. part-skim mozzarella cheese, shredded
- 4 tbsps fresh basil leaves, chopped
- 4 large egg whites
- Freshly ground black pepper, to taste
- 6 cups cooked whole-wheat spaghetti
- 0.6 cup scallion, chopped
- 8 large eggs
- 10 cups fat-free milk

Directions:

- In a bowl, add eggs, egg whites, and black pepper and beat until well combined.
- Set aside.
- In a medium non-stick skillet, heat oil over medium heat.
- In the bottom of the skillet, place the spaghetti evenly and cook for about 2 minutes.
- Top with egg mixture evenly and sprinkle with cheese, scallion, and basil.

- Cook, covered for about 8 minutes.
- Remove from the heat and cut into 4 equal-sized wedges and serve.

4 Serving

Preparation time: 31 minutes

Ingredients:

- 0.25 tsp. ground cumin
- Freshly ground black pepper, to taste
- 6 garlic cloves, minced
- 1 cup onion, chopped
- 2 small tomato, chopped
- 8 egg whites
- Pinch of salt
- 2 tbsps. olive oil
- 4 tbsps. green chili, chopped
- 4 cups zucchini, sliced thinly
- 4 tsps. fresh parsley, chopped
- 4 large eggs

Directions:

- In a bowl, add eggs, egg whites, and spices and beat until well combined. Set aside.
- In a 12-inch non-stick skillet, heat oil over medium heat and sauté onion for about 2 minutes. Add garlic and green chili and sauté for about 1 mintute.
- Add zucchini and sauté for about 2-3 minutes. Sprinkle with tomato and parsley

and immediately top with egg mixture
evenly.
- Reduce the heat to low and cook, covered
  for about 10 minutes. Remove from the
  heat and cut into 4 equal-sized portions
  and serve.

LUNCH

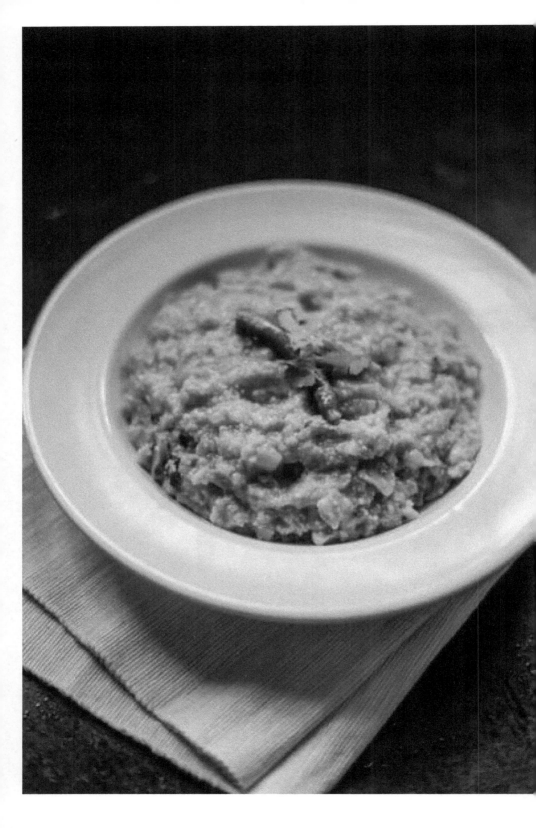

Lentil & Spinach Chili

16 Serving

Preparation time: 2 hours, 35 minutes

Ingredients:

- 1 tbsp. dried thyme, crushed
- 1 tbsp. cayenne pepper
- 6 tbsps. ground cumin
- Freshly ground black pepper, to taste
- 2 lb. lentils, rinsed
- 12 cups fresh spinach
- 2 large onion, chopped
- 8 celery stalks, chopped
- 2 jalapeño pepper, seeded and chopped
- 2 tbsps. chipotle chili powder
- 6 tbsps. ground coriander
- 2 tsps. ground turmeric
- 4 tbsps. salt-free tomato paste
- 16 cups low-sodium vegetable broth
- 1 cup fresh cilantro, chopped
- 4 tsps. olive oil
- 6 medium carrot, peeled and chopped
- 4 garlic cloves, minced

Directions:

- In a large pan, heat oil over medium heat and sauté onion for about 4-5 minutes. Add carrot and celery for about 5 minutes. Add garlic, jalapeño pepper, thyme, and spices and sauté for about 1 minute.

- Add tomato paste, lentils, and broth and bring to a boil.
- Reduce the heat to low and simmer, partially covered for about 2 hours.
- Stir in spinach and simmer for about 3-4 minutes.
- Serve hot with the garnishing of cilantro.

Lentil Curry

6 Serving

Preparation time: 1 hour 20 minutes

Ingredients:

- 2 tbsps. ground turmeric
- 2 cups dried brown lentils
- 6 cups water
- 2 (30-oz.) can coconut milk
- 2 tbsps. cumin seeds
- 2 head garlic, peeled and chopped
- 4 tbsps. fresh ginger, chopped
- Pinch of salt
- 2-4 tsps. cayenne pepper
- 1 cup fresh cilantro, chopped
- 2 tbsps. olive oil
- 2 tbsps. coriander seeds
- 6-8 cups tomatoes, chopped finely

Directions:

- In a large pan, melt the coconut oil over medium-high heat and toast the cumin and coriander seeds for about 45 seconds, stirring continuously.
- Add the garlic and sauté for about 2 minutes. Add the tomatoes, ginger, turmeric and salt and cook for about 5 minutes, stirring continuously. Add the lentils, water and

cayenne pepper and bring to a boil. Reduce the heat to low and simmer, covered for about 35-40 minutes, stirring occasionally.

- Add the coconut milk and stir to combine. Increase the heat to medium and bring to a boil. Remove from the heat and stir in the cilantro. Serve hot.

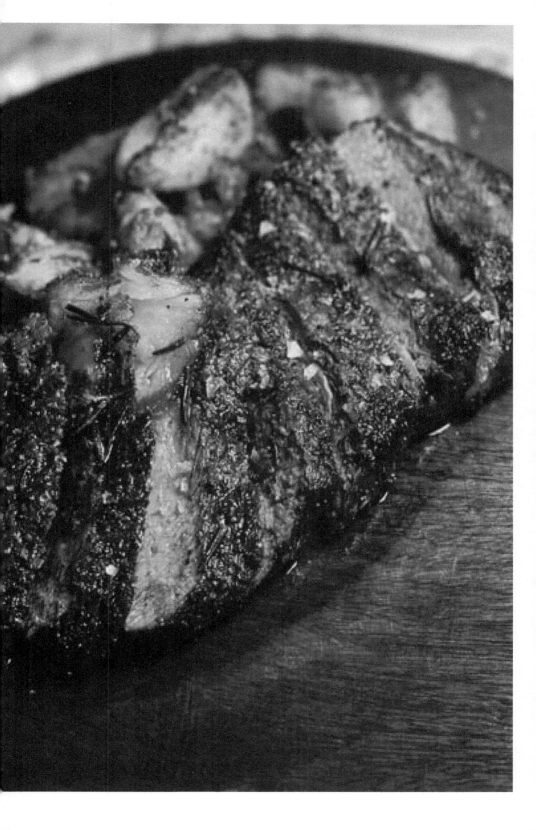

Ground Beef with Lentils

6 Servings

Preparation Time: 10 hour and 5 minutes

Ingredients

- 3 tablespoons extra-virgin olive oil, divided.
- 1 tablespoon fresh ginger, minced.
- 2 cups dried red lentils, soaked for 30 minutes, and drained.
- 2 teaspoons cumin seeds
- half teaspoons cayenne pepper
- 1 onion, chopped.
- 4 garlic cloves, minced.
- 3 plum tomatoes, chopped. finely
- 2 cups low-sodium chicken broth
- 1 lb. lean ground beef
- 1 jalapeño pepper seeded and chopped.

Directions:

- In a Dutch oven, heat 1 tablespoons of oil over medium heat and sauté the onion, ginger, and garlic for about 5 minutes.
- Stir in the tomatoes, lentils and broth and bring to a boil.
- Reduce the heat to medium-low and simmer, covered for about 30 minutes.

- Meanwhile, in a skillet, heat the remaining oil over medium heat.
- Add the cumin seeds and sauté for about 30 seconds.
- Add the paprika and sauté for about 30 seconds.
- Pour the mixture into a small bowl and set aside.
- In the same skillet, add the beef and cook for about 4-5 minutes.
- Add jalapeño and scallion and cook for about 4-5 minutes.
- Add the spiced oil mixture and stir to combine well.
- Pour the beef mixture into the simmering lentils and simmer for about 10-15 minutes or until desired doneness. Serve hot.

Ground Beef with Barley

4 Servings

Preparation Time: 1 hour and 20 minutes

Ingredients

- 1 cupwater
- 2 teaspoons extra-virgin olive oil
- 1 cupfresh mushrooms, sliced.
- 2 cups frozen green beans
- Freshly ground black pepper, to taste
- quarter cuppearl barley
- 7 oz. lean ground beef
- ¾ cuponion, chopped.
- quarter cuplow-sodium beef broth
- 2 tablespoons fresh parsley, chopped.

Directions:

- In a pan, add water and barley over medium heat and bring to a boil.
- Reduce the heat to low and simmer, covered for about 30-40 minutes or until all the liquid is absorbed.
- Remove from heat and set aside.
- In a skillet, heat oil over medium-high heat and cook beef for about 8-10 minutes.

- Add mushroom and onion and cook for about 5-6 minutes.
- Add green beans and cook for about 2-3 minutes.
- Stir in cooked barley, broth, and soy sauce and cook for about 3-4 minutes more.
- Stir in parsley and serve hot.

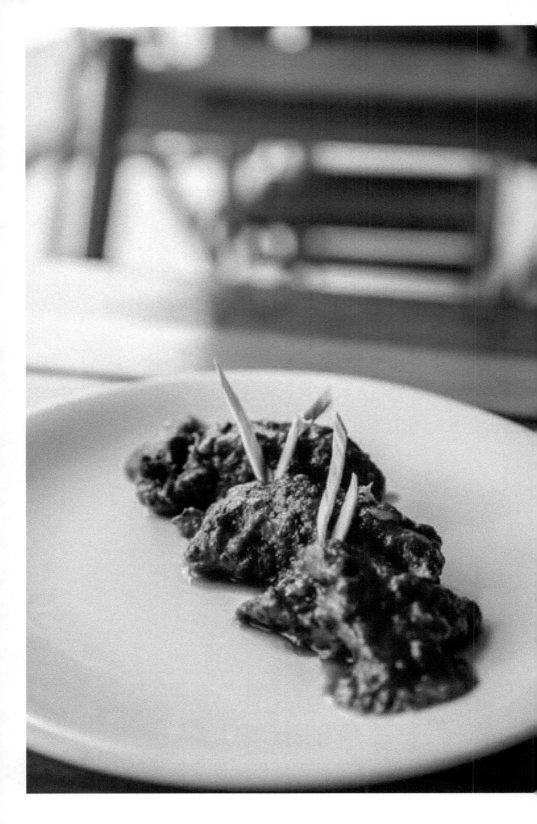

6 Servings

Preparation time: 45 minutes

Ingredients:

- 1 teaspoon chili powder
- 1 ½teaspoon sweet paprika
- 1 garlic clove, minced
- 1 ½yellow onion, chopped
- 1½ big turkey breast, skinless, boneless, and cubed
- 1½ cuplow-sodium chicken stock
- 1 ½tablespoon coconut oil, melted
- 1 ½Savoy cabbage, shredded
-

Directions:

- Heat up a pan with the oil over medium heat, add the meat, and brown for 5 minutes.
- Add the garlic and the onion, toss and sauté for 5 minutes more.
- Add the cabbage and the other ingredients, toss, bring to a simmer and cook over medium heat for 25 minutes.
- Divide everything between plates and serve.

6 Servings

Preparation time: 40 minutes

Ingredients:

- 1 tablespoon ginger, grated
- 1 teaspoon oregano, dried
- 1 teaspoon cumin, ground
- 1½ teaspoon allspice, ground
- 1 cupcilantro, chopped
- A pinch of black pepper
- 1 pound chicken breast, skinless, boneless, and sliced
- 6 scallions, chopped
- 1½ tablespoon olive oil
- 1½ tablespoon sweet paprika
- 1 cuplow-sodium chicken stock
-

Directions:

- Heat up a pan with the oil over medium heat, add the scallions and the meat, and brown for 5 minutes.

- Add the rest of the ingredients, toss, introduce in the oven and bake at 390 degrees F for 25 minutes.
- Divide the chicken and scallions, mix between plates and serve.

6 Servings

Preparation time: 45minutes

Ingredients:

- 1½ shallot, chopped
- 1 cuplow-sodium chicken stock
- 3 garlic cloves, minced
- 1 teaspoon basil, dried
- 1 pound chicken thighs, boneless and skinless
- 1 tablespoon avocado oil
- 2 tablespoons mustard
-

Directions:

- Heat up a pan with the oil over medium heat, add the shallot, garlic, and the chicken, and brown everything for 5 minutes.
- Add the mustard and the rest of the ingredients, toss gently, bring to a simmer and cook over medium heat for 30 minutes.
- Divide everything between plates and serve hot.

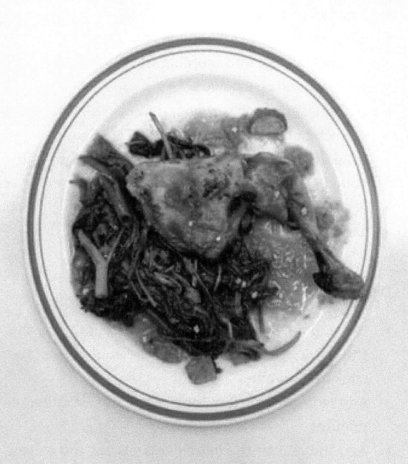

6 Servings

Preparation time: 45 minutes

Ingredients:

- 3 garlic cloves, minced
- 1½ poblano pepper, chopped
- 1½ cuplow-sodium vegetable stock
- 1½ teaspoon chili powder
- 2 ½tablespoons chives, chopped
- A pinch of black pepper
- 2½ pounds chicken breast, skinless, boneless, and cubed
- 2 ½tablespoons olive oil
- 1½ cupcelery, chopped

Directions:

- Heat up a pan with the oil over medium heat, add the garlic, celery, and poblano pepper, toss and cook for 5 minutes.
- Add the meat, toss and cook for another 5 minutes.
- Add the rest of the ingredients except the chives, bring to a simmer and cook over medium heat for 25 minutes more.

- Divide the whole mix between plates and serve with the chives sprinkled on top.

Chicken & Strawberry Salad

16 Servings

Preparation time: 36 minutes

Ingredients:

- 2 garlic clove, minced
- Freshly ground black pepper, to taste
- 16 cups fresh spinach, torn
- 1 cup olive oil
- 4 tbsps. Erythritol
- Pinch of salt
- 8 cups fresh strawberries
- 4 lbs boneless, skinless chicken breasts
- 0.5 cup fresh lemon juice

Directions:

- For the marinade: in a large bowl, add oil, lemon juice, Erythritol, garlic, salt, and black pepper, and beat until well combined. In a large resealable plastic bag, place chicken and ¾ CUPmarinade.
- Seal bag and shake to coat well. Refrigerate overnight. Cover the bowl of remaining marinade and refrigerate before serving. Preheat the grill to medium heat. Grease the grill grate. Remove the chicken from the bag and discard the marinade.

Place the chicken onto grill grate and grill, covered for about 5-8 minutes per side.
- Remove chicken from grill and cut into bite-sized pieces.
- In a large bowl, add the chicken pieces, strawberries, and spinach, and mix. Place the reserved marinade and toss to coat. Serve immediately.

8 Servings

Preparation time: 18 minutes

Ingredients:

- 2 tbsps. Dijon mustard
- 2 garlic cloves, minced
- Freshly ground black pepper, to taste
- 6 cups apples, cored and sliced thinly
- 1 cup fresh mint leaves, chopped
- 0.5 cup olive oil
- 2 tbsps. unsweetened applesauce
- Pinch of salt
- 4 tbsps. fresh cilantro, chopped
- 24 medium shrimp
- 6 cups carrot, peeled and julienned
- 4 tbsps. organic apple cider vinegar

Directions:

- In a large pan of boiling water, add shrimp and cook for about 3 minutes.
- Drain the shrimp well and set aside to cool. After cooling, peel and devein the shrimps.
- In a large bowl, add cooked shrimp and remaining all ingredients except cilantro and gently stir to combine.
- Cover and refrigerate to chill for about 1 hour. Top with cilantro and serve.

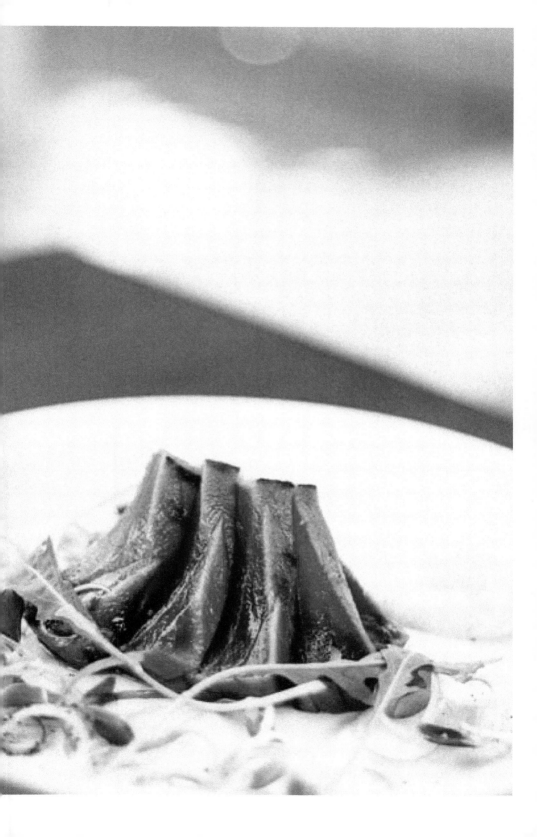

SNACKS

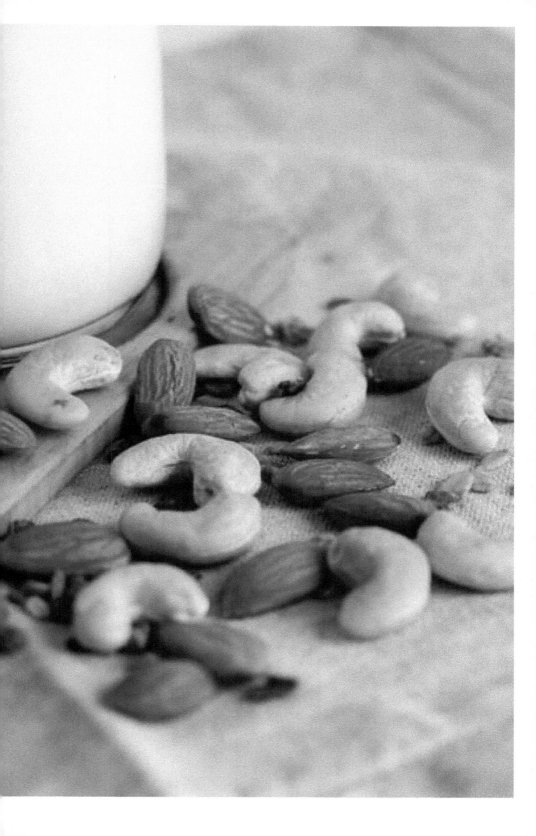

24 Servings

Preparation time: 20 minutes

Ingredients:

- 0.5 tsp. cayenne pepper
- 1 tsp. ground cumin
- 2 tbsps. fresh lemon juice
- 4 cups raw unsalted cashews

Directions:

- Preheat the oven to 400 °F. Line a large roasting pan with a piece of foil.
- In a large bowl, add the cashews and spices and toss to coat well. Transfer the cashews into the prepared roasting pan. Roast for about 8-10 minutes. Drizzle with lemon juice and serve.

30 Servings

Preparation time: 10 minutes

Ingredients

- 4 seedless navel oranges, cut into thin slices

Directions

- Set the dehydrator on 135 °F.
- Arrange the orange slices onto the dehydrator sheets.
- Dehydrate for about 10 hours.

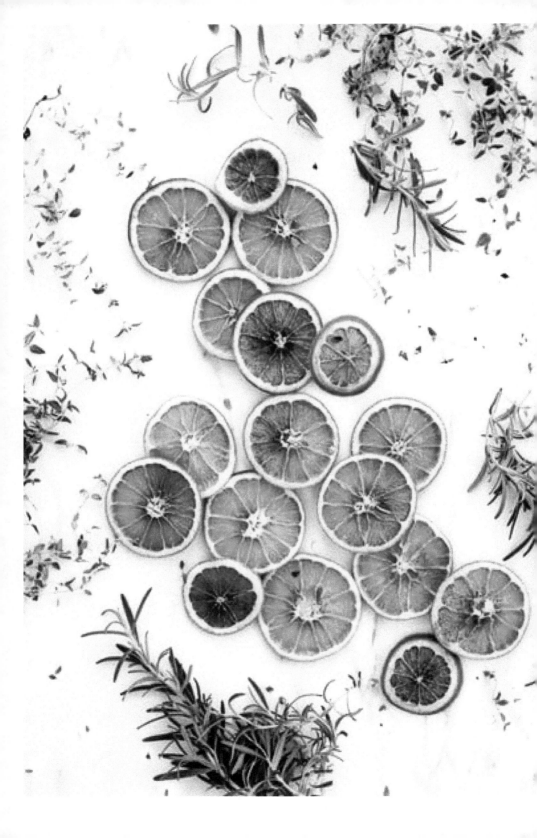

12 Servings

Preparation time: 25 minutes

Ingredients

- 0.5 tsp. cayenne pepper

- 2 lbs. fresh kale leaves, tough ribs removed and torn
- 2 tbsps. olive oil

Directions

- Preheat the oven to 35o °F.
- Line a large baking sheet with parchment paper.
- Arrange the kale pieces onto the prepared baking sheet in a single layer. Sprinkle the kale with cayenne pepper and drizzle with oil. Bake for 10-15 minutes.
- Remove from the oven and let the chips cool before serving.

8 Servings

Preparation time: 1 hour, 10 minutes

Ingredients:

- 2 large bananas, peeled

Directions:

- Prepare the oven to 250 °F.
- Line a large baking sheet with baking paper.
- Cut each banana into ¼-inch thick slices.
- Place the banana slices onto the prepared baking sheet in a single layer.
- Bake for about 1 hour.
- Remove from the oven and let the chips cool before serving.

Devilled Eggs

12 Servings

Preparation time: 20 minutes

Ingredients:

- 2medium avocado, peeled, pitted, and chopped
- Pinch of cayenne pepper
- 12 large eggs
- 4 tsps. fresh lime juice
- Pinch of salt

Directions:

- In a large pan of water, add the eggs and bring to a boil over high heat.
- Cover the pan and immediately remove it from the heat.
- Set aside, covered for at least 10-15 minutes.
- Drain the eggs and let them cool completely. Peel the eggs and, with a sharp knife, slice them in half vertically. Remove the yolks from egg halves. In a bowl, add half of the egg yolks, avocado, lime juice, and a Pinch of salt with a fork, mash until well combined. Scoop the avocado mixture into the egg halves evenly. Serve with a sprinkling of cayenne pepper.

Sweet Potato Fries

4 Servings

Preparation time: 35 minutes

Ingredients:

- 4 tbsps. extra-virgin olive oil
- 2 tsps. ground turmeric
- 2 tsps. ground cinnamon
- Freshly ground black pepper, to taste
- 2 large sweet potato, peeled and cut into wedges
- Pinch of salt

Directions:

- Preheat the oven to 425 °F. Line a baking sheet with foil paper. In a large bowl, add all ingredients and toss to coat well. Transfer the sweet potato wedges onto the prepared baking sheet and spread them into an even layer. Bake for 25 minutes, flipping once after 15 minutes. Remove from the oven and serve immediately.

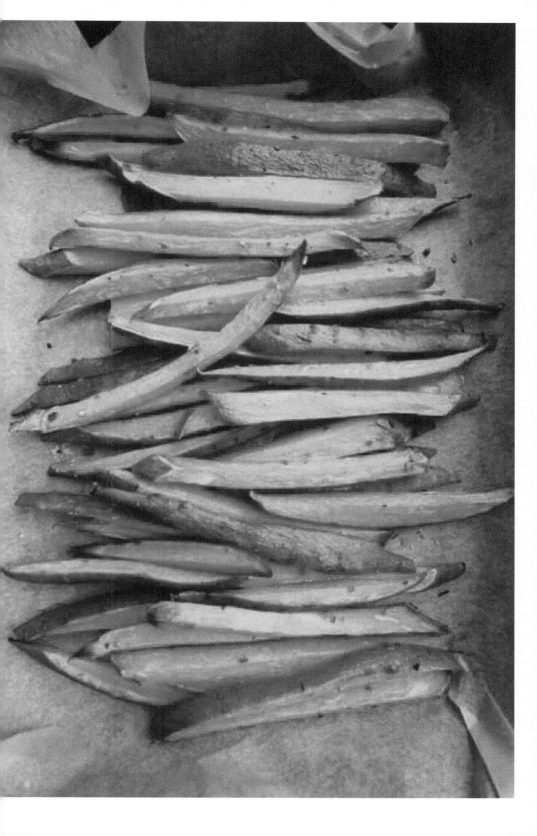

Mixed Fruit Bowl

12 Servings

Preparation time: 15 minutes

Ingredients:

- 4 tbsps. almonds, chopped
- 1 cupfresh strawberries, hulled and sliced
- 1 cup fresh cherries pitted and halved
- 2 tbsps. fresh lemon juice
- 2 cups banana, peeled and sliced
- 1 cup fresh blueberries
- 4 tbsps. maple syrup

Directions:

- In a large bowl, add fruit, maple syrup, and lemon juice and gently toss to coat well.
- Place fruit mixture into serving bowls.
- Top with almonds and serve.

4 Servings

Preparation time: 50 minutes

Ingredients:

- 4 large apples
- ¾ cuppecans, chopped
- 1 tsp. ground cinnamon
- 1/8 tsp. ground allspice
- ¾ cup water
- ¾ cup oats
- 3 tbsps. unsweetened applesauce
- ¼ tsp. ground ginger

Directions:

- Preheat the oven to 350 °F. In a bowl, mix together the oats, pecans, applesauce, and spices.
- Set aside. Remove the top of each apple. With a spoon, carefully scoop out the flesh from inside of the apples.
- Stuff the apples with pecan mixture evenly. Arrange the apples into a baking dish. Add water to the baking dish. Bake for about 30-40 minutes. Serve warm.

DINNER

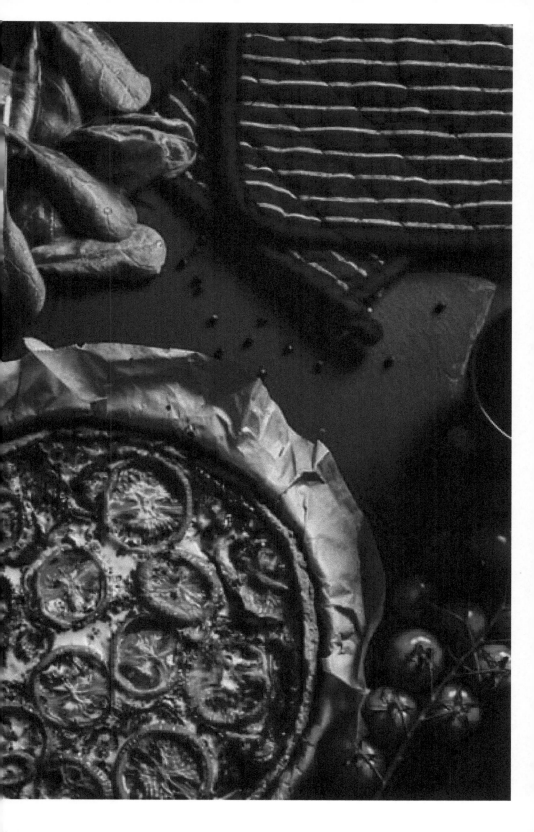

12 Servings

Preparation time: 15 minutes and 1¼ hours

Ingredients:

- 4 medium zucchinis, chopped
- 6 cups cooked red kidney beans
- 4 cups low-sodium vegetable broth
- 2 medium onions, chopped
- 2 tsps. ground cumin
- 2 tbsps. red chili powder
- 2 large bell pepper, seeded and chopped
- 6 cups tomatoes, chopped
- 6 cups cooked white beans
- 0.5 cup fresh cilantro leaves, chopped
- 4 tbsps. olive oil
- 8 garlic cloves, minced
- 0.5 tsp. ground coriander
- Freshly ground black pepper, to taste

Directions:

- In a Dutch oven, heat the oil over medium heat and cook the onion for about 8-9 minutes, stirring frequently.
- Add the garlic, spices, and black pepper and sauté for about 1 minute.
- Add the remaining ingredients except for cilantro and bring to a boil. Reduce the heat to

low and simmer, covered for about 1 hour. Serve hot with the garnishing of cilantro.

Beans & Mushroom Chili

4 Servings

Preparation time: 1 hour 40 minutes

Ingredients:

- 1 tbsps. ground cumin
- 8 oz. cooked kidney beans
- 2 cups tomatoes, chopped finely
- 1 medium onion, chopped
- 1 small bell pepper, seeded and chopped
- 2 garlic cloves, minced
- 1 tbsps. red chili powder
- Freshly ground black pepper, to taste
- 8 oz. cooked white kidney beans
- 1½ cup low-sodium vegetable broth
- 2 tbsps. avocado oil
- 1 carrot, peeled and chopped
- 1 lbs. fresh mushrooms, sliced
- 2 tsps. dried oregano

Directions:

- In a large Dutch oven, heat the oil over medium-low heat and cook the onions, carrot, and bell pepper for about 10 minutes, stirring frequently.
- Reduce the heat to medium-high. Stir in the mushrooms and garlic and cook for about 5-6 minutes, stirring frequently. Add the oregano,

spices, salt, and black pepper, and cook for about 1-2 minutes.

- Stir in the beans, tomatoes, and broth and bring to a boil.
- Reduce the heat to low and simmer, covered for about 1 hour, stirring occasionally. Serve hot.

Cod in Lemon Sauce

4 Servings

Preparation time: 23 minutes

Ingredients:

- Pinch of salt
- 6 tbsps. olive oil, divided
- 2-4 lemon slices
- 4 (12-oz.) cod fillets
- Freshly ground black pepper, to taste
- 4 garlic cloves, minced
- 4 tsps. fresh dill weed

Directions:

- Season each cod fillet evenly with salt and black pepper. In a medium skillet, heat 1 tbsp. of oil over high heat and cook the cod fillets for about 4-5 minutes per side.
- Transfer the cod fillets onto a plate. Meanwhile, in a frying pan, heat the remaining oil over low heat and sauté the garlic and lemon slices for about 40-60 seconds.
- Stir in the cooked cod fillets and dill and cook, covered for about 1-2 minutes. Remove the cod fillets from heat and transfer them onto the serving plates.
- Top with the pan sauce and serve immediately

Sardine with Olives

4 Servings

Preparation time: 30 minutes

Ingredients:
- 4 tbsps olive oil
- 4 cups fresh parsley leaves, chopped
- 4 tbsps. capers, drained
- 4 Serrano peppers, seeded and minced
- 24 (4-oz.) fresh sardines, cleaned and scaled
- Freshly ground black pepper, to taste
- 1 cupgreen olives, pitted and chopped
- 2 tbsps. fresh oregano, chopped
- 4 garlic cloves, thinly sliced
- 2 tsps. fresh lemon zest, grated finely
- Pinch of salt

Directions:
- Preheat the oven to 400 °F. Season the sardines with salt and black pepper lightly.
- In a large ovenproof skillet, heat the oil over medium heat and cook the sardines for about 3 minutes.
- Flip the sardines and stir in the remaining ingredients.

- Immediately, transfer the skillet into the oven and bake for about 5 minutes or until the desired doneness of the fish.
- Remove from oven and serve hot

Baked Beef & Veggies Stew

16 Servings

Preparation time: 15 minutes and 3 hours

Ingredients:
- 4 medium onion, chopped
- 2 tbsps. fresh thyme, chopped
- 4 cups low-sodium chicken broth
- 6 tbsps. arrowroot starch
- 2 lbs. fresh mushrooms, sliced
- 8 medium carrots, peeled and chopped
- 4 celery stalks, chopped
- 4 garlic cloves, minced
- Freshly ground black pepper, to taste
- 2 cups water
- 2 (4-lb.) beef chuck roast, trimmed and cubed
- 4 cups tomatoes, chopped

Directions:
- Preheat the oven to 325 °F.
- In a bowl, mix together water and arrowroot starch.
- In a large ovenproof pan, add remaining ingredients and stir to combine.
- Slowly add arrowroot starch mixture, stirring continuously.
- Cover the pan and bake for about 3 hours, stirring after every 30 minutes. Serve hot.

Shrimp Stew

12 Servings

Preparation time: 35 minutes

Ingredients

- 4 tbsps fresh lime juice
- 1 cuponion, chopped finely
- 2 Serrano pepper, chopped
- 8 cups fresh tomatoes, chopped
- 4 lb. shrimp, peeled and deveined
- 4 tbsps. fresh basil, chopped
- 4 tbsps. olive oil
- 4 garlic cloves, minced
- 2 tsps smoked paprika
- 6 cups low-sodium chicken broth

Directions:

- In a large soup pan, heat oil over medium-high heat and sauté the onion for about 5-6 minutes.
- Add the garlic, Serrano pepper, and paprika and sauté for about 1 minute.
- Add the tomatoes and broth and bring to a boil.
- Reduce the heat to medium and simmer for about 5 minutes.
- Stir in the shrimp and cook for about 4-5 minutes.
- Stir in lemon juice and basil and remove from heat.Serve hot.

Sea-Food Stew

16 Servings

Preparation time: 50 minutes

Ingredients:

- 0.5 tsp. red pepper flakes, crushed
- 6 cups low-sodium fish broth
- 1 lb. shrimp, peeled and deveined
- 0.5 lb. bay scallops
- 4 tbsps fresh lemon juice
- 2 medium yellow onion, chopped
- 2 jalapeño pepper, chopped
- lb. fresh tomatoes, chopped
- 2 lb. red snapper fillets, cubed
- 0.5 lb. fresh squid, cleaned and cut into rings
- 0.5 lb. mussels
- 1 cup fresh parsley, chopped
- 4 tbsps olive oil
- 6 garlic cloves, minced

Directions:

- In a large soup pan, heat oil over medium heat and sauté the onion for about 5-6 minutes. Add the garlic, Serrano pepper, and red pepper flakes and sauté for about 1 minute.
- Add tomatoes and broth and bring to a gentle simmer. Reduce the heat to low and cook for about 10 minutes.

- Add the snapper and cook for about 2 minutes. Stir in the remaining seafood and cook for about 6-8 minutes.
- Stir in the lemon juice, basil, salt, and black pepper, and remove from heat. Serve hot.

6 Servings

Preparation time: 50 minutes

Ingredients:

- 1 teaspoon chili powder
- 1½ teaspoon rosemary, dried
- 2 cups low-sodium chicken stock
- A pinch of black pepper
- Zest of 1 lime, grated
- 1 tablespoon lime juice
- 1½ tablespoon cilantro, chopped
- 1 ½turkey breast, skinless, boneless, and sliced
- 2 tablespoons olive oil
- 1 pound baby potatoes, peeled and halved
- 1 ½tablespoon sweet paprika
- 1½ yellow onion, chopped

Directions:

- Heat up a pan with the oil over medium heat, add the onion, chili powder, and rosemary, toss and sauté for 5 minutes.
- Add the meat, and brown for 5 minutes more.

- Add the potatoes and the rest of the ingredients except the cilantro toss gently, bring to a simmer and cook over medium heat for 30 minutes.
- Divide the mix between plates and serve with the cilantro sprinkled on top.

DESSERT

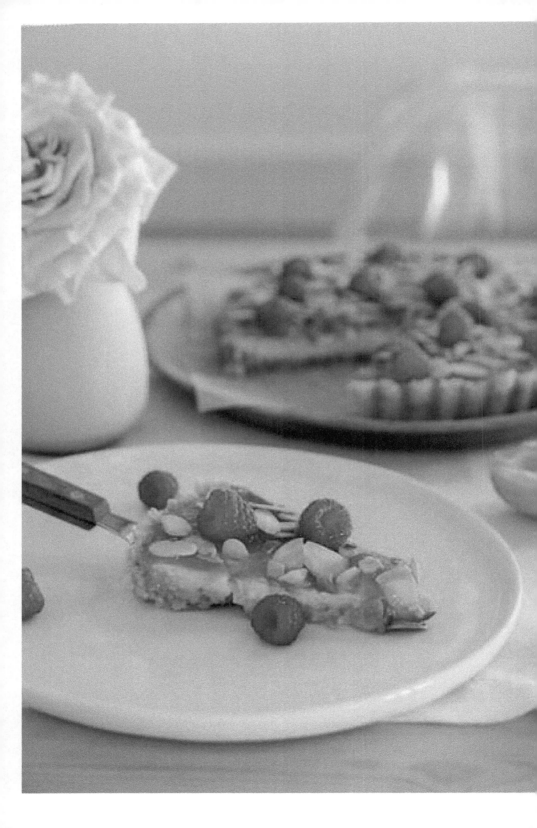

Chocolate Tofu Mousse

12 Servings

Preparation time: 15 minutes

Ingredients:

- 0.5 cupunsweetened almond milk
- 20-30 drops liquid stevia
- 0.5 cup fresh strawberries
- 2 lb. firm tofu, pressed and drained
- 4 tbsps. cacao powder
- 2 tbsps. organic vanilla extract

Directions:

- In a blender, add all ingredients except the strawberries and pulse until creamy and smooth.
- Transfer into serving bowls and refrigerate to chill for at least 2 hours. Garnish with strawberries and serve.

8 Serving

Preparation time: 10 minutes

Ingredients:

- 1 cupunsweetened almond milk
- 8 Medjool dates, pitted and chopped
- 4 tbsps. cacao powder
- 8 tbsps. fresh blueberries
- 2 cups cooked black beans
- 1 cuppecans, chopped
- 2 tsps. organic vanilla extract

Directions:

- In a food processor, add all the ingredients and pulse until smooth and creamy.
- Transfer the mixture into serving bowls and refrigerate to chill before serving. Garnish with blueberries and serve.

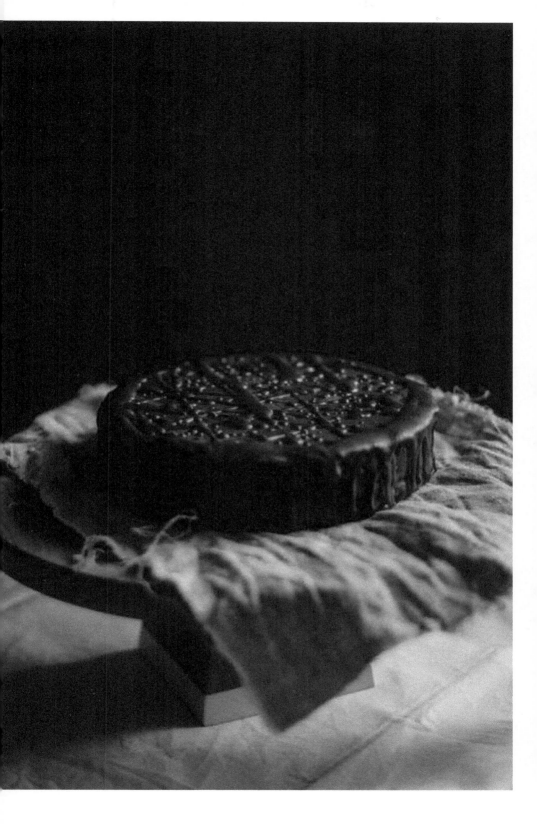

8 Servings

Preparation time: 15 minutes

Ingredients:

- 2 tsps fresh lime zest, grated finely
- 1 cup fresh lime juice
- 0.6 cup unsweetened applesauce
- 4 avocados, peeled, pitted, and chopped
- 2 tsps fresh lemon zest, grated finely
- 1 cup fresh lemon juice
- 4 cups bananas, peeled and chopped

Directions:

- In a blender, add all the ingredients and pulse until smooth.
- Transfer into 4 serving glasses and refrigerate to chill for about 3 hours before serving.

Strawberry Soufflé

12 Servings

Preparation time: 32 minutes

Ingredients:

- 0.6 cup unsweetened applesauce, divided
- 8 tsps. fresh lemon juice
- 36 oz. fresh strawberries, hulled
- 10 egg whites, divided

Directions:

- Preheat the oven to 350 °F. In a blender, ad strawberries and pulse until pureed. Through a strainer, strain the strawberry puree in a bowl and discard the seeds.
- In the bowl of strawberry puree, add 3 tbsps of applesauce, 2 egg whites, and lemon juice and beat until frothy and light.
- In another bowl, add remaining egg whites and beat until frothy. While beating gradually, add remaining applesauce and beat until stiff peaks form. Gently fold the egg whites into strawberry mixture.
- Transfer the mixture into 6 large ramekins evenly. Arrange the ramekins onto a baking sheet. Bake for about 10-12 minutes. Serve warm.

Beans Brownies

24 Servings

Preparation time: 45 minutes

Ingredients:

- 4 tsps organic vanilla extract
- 2 tbsps ground cinnamon
- 24 Medjool dates, pitted and chopped
- 4 tbsps quick rolled oats
- 0.5CUP cacao powder
- 4 cups cooked black beans
- 4 tbsps almond butter

Directions:

- Preheat the oven to 350 °F. Line a large baking dish with parchment paper. In a food processor, add all the ingredients except the cacao powder and cinnamon and pulse until well combined and smooth.
- Transfer the mixture into a large bowl. Add the cacao powder and cinnamon and stir to combine. Now, transfer the mixture into the prepared baking dish evenly, and with the back of a spatula, smooth the top surface.
- Bake for about 30 minutes. Remove from oven and place onto a wire rack to cool completely.

With a sharp knife, cut into 12 equal-sized brownies and serve.

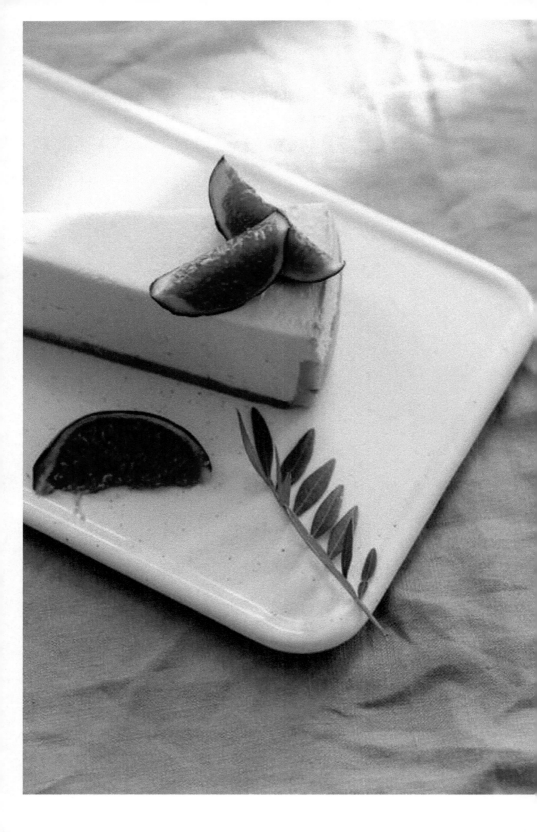

Chocolate Cupcakes

12 Servings

Preparation time: 30 minutes

Ingredients:

- 2 tbsps organic baking powder
- 0.5 cups unsweetened almond milk
- 2 cups dates pitted
- 0.6 cup cacao powder
- Pinch of salt
- 2 cups water
- 2 cups oat flour

Directions:

- Preheat the oven to 350 °F. Line 6 cups of a muffin tin with paper liners. In a food processor, add water and dates and pulse until smooth.
- In a large bowl, mix together flour, cacao powder, baking powder, and salt. Add the almond milk and date paste and beat until well combined. Transfer the mixture into paper muffin cups.
- Bake for 25 minutes or until a toothpick inserted in the center comes out clean. Remove the muffin tin from the oven and place it onto a wire rack to cool for about 10 minutes. Carefully invert the cupcakes onto a wire rack to cool completely before serving.

10 Servings

Preparation time: 65 minutes

Ingredients:

- 12 whole-wheat bread slices
- 2 cups apple, peeled, cored, and cut into ½-inch pieces
- 1 cup raisins
- 6 cups fresh apple juice
- 1 tsp. stevia
- 4tbsps. unsalted margarine softened
- 2 cups mango, peeled, pitted, and cut into ½-inch pieces
- 1 cup dried apricots, chopped into small pieces
- 1 cup unsalted walnuts, chopped
- 1 tsp. ground cinnamon

Directions:

- Preheat the oven to 350 °F. Lightly grease a 9X9-inch baking dish. Spread margarine over bread slices lightly.
- Cut each bread slice into 1-inch pieces. In a large bowl, mix together bread pieces, mangos, apples, apricots, raisins, and walnuts. In a small bowl, mix together apple juice, cinnamon, and stevia.

- Place the juice mixture over the bread mixture and mix all. Place the bread mixture into the prepared baking dish evenly.
- With a piece of foil, cover the baking dish. Bake for about 30 minutes.
- Uncover and bake for about 20 minutes or until the top becomes golden brown.
- Serve warm.

Blackberry Crumble

8 Servings

Preparation time: 50 minutes

Ingredients:
- 6 tbsp. water
- 0.5 cup arrowroot flour
- 4 tbsps. olive oil
- 1 tbsp. fresh lemon juice
- 6 cups fresh blackberries
- 0.5 cupcoconut flour
- 1.5 tsps baking soda
- 0.5 cup banana, peeled and mashed

Directions:
- Preheat the oven to 300 °F. Lightly grease an 8x8-inch baking dish. In a large bowl, mix together all ingredients except blackberries. Place blackberries in the bottom of the prepared baking dish.
- Spread flour mixture over blackberries evenly. Bake for 35-40 minutes or until the top becomes golden brown. Serve warm.

Strawberry Crumb

8 Servings

Preparation time: 40 minutes

Ingredients

- 0.5 tsp. ground cinnamon
- 2 tsps arrowroot starch
- 4 tbsps almond flour
- 4 tbsps pecans, chopped
- 6 cups fresh strawberries, hulled and chopped
- 1 cup oat flour
- 6 tbsp. almond butter

Directions:

- Preheat the oven to 350 °F. For filling: in a baking dish, place strawberries and arrowroot starch and gently mix. For the topping: in a bowl, add remaining ingredients and mix until a crumbly mixture forms.
- Spread the topping over strawberries evenly. Bake for about 20-25 minutes or until the top becomes golden brown. Serve warm.

SALADS AND SOUPS

16 Servings

Preparation time: 36 minutes

Ingredients:

- 2 garlic clove, minced
- Freshly ground black pepper, to taste
- 16 cups fresh spinach, torn
- 1 cup olive oil
- 4 tbsps Erythritol
- Pinch of salt
- 8 cups of fresh strawberries
- 4 lb boneless, skinless chicken breasts
- 0.5 cup fresh lemon juice

Directions:

- For the marinade: in a large bowl, add oil, lemon juice, Erythritol, garlic, salt, and black pepper, and beat until well combined. In a large resealable plastic bag, place chicken and ¾ cup marinade.
- Seal bag and shake to coat well. Refrigerate overnight. Cover the bowl of remaining marinade and refrigerate before serving— Preheat the grill to medium heat.
- Grease the grill grate. Remove the chicken from bag and discard the marinade. Place

the chicken onto grill grate and grill, covered for about 5-8 minutes per side.

- Remove chicken from grill and cut into bite-sized pieces.
- In a large bowl, add the chicken pieces, strawberries and spinach and mix.
- Place the reserved marinade and toss to coat.
- Serve immediately.

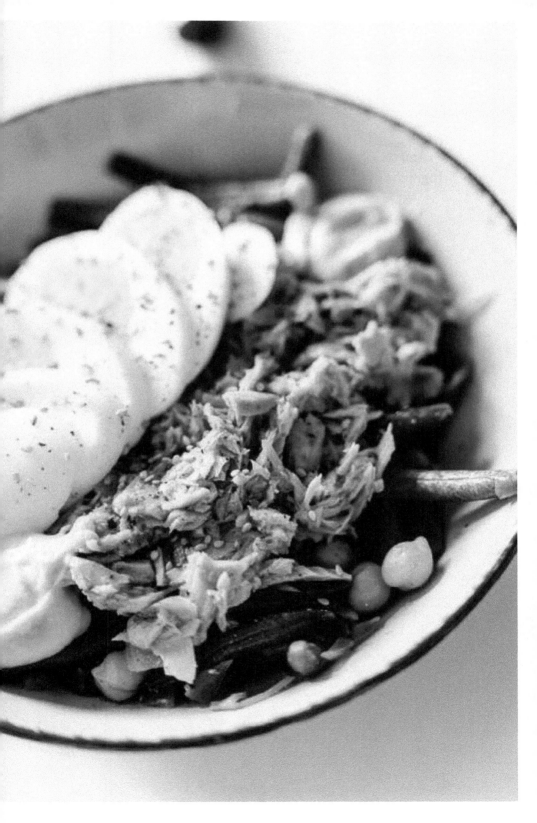

Beef & Cabbage Salad

4 Servings

Preparation time: 15 minutes
Ingredients:

- 2 cups cabbage, shredded
- 2 large tomato, chopped
- 6 tbsp. feta cheese, crumbled
- 12 oz. cooked lean beef, chopped
- 2 cups cooked chickpeas
- 2 tbsps balsamic vinegar
- Freshly ground black pepper, to taste
- 2 tbsps olive oil
- 0.25 tsp. red pepper flakes, crushed
- 0.5 tsp. dried basil

Directions:

- In a large bowl, add all ingredients except for feta cheese and mix.
- In a small bowl, add all ingredients and beat until well combined. Add dressing in the bowl of salad and gently toss to coat well.
- Serve immediately with the topping of feta cheese.

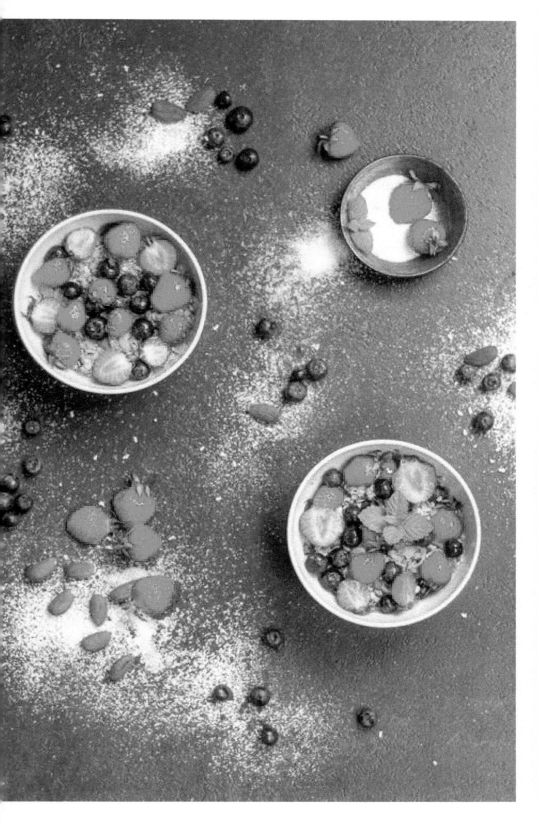

12 Servings

Preparation time: 15 minutes

Ingredients:

- 2 cups fresh strawberries, hulled and sliced
- 2 tsps unsalted cashews, chopped
- 6 tsps olive oil
- 4 cups cucumbers, sliced
- 2 cups cherry tomatoes, halved
- 4 cups romaine lettuce, torn
- 4 tbsps. fresh lemon juice
- 32 oz. water-packed tuna chunks, drained
- 2 cups fresh mushrooms, sliced

Directions:

- In a large serving bowl, add all ingredients and gently toss to coat well.
- Serve immediately.

12 Servings

Preparation time: 21 minutes

Ingredients:

- Pinch of salt
- 8 cups fresh arugula
- 4 tbsps olive oil
- 2 garlic clove, crushed and divided
- 2 lb. shrimp, peeled and deveined
- Freshly ground black pepper, to taste
- 4 cups lettuce, torn
- 4 tbsps fresh lime juice
- 2 tbsps olive oil
- 4 tbsps fresh rosemary, chopped

Directions:

- In a large skillet, heat the oil over medium heat and sauté garlic for about 1 minute. Add the shrimp with salt and black pepper and cook for about 4-5 minutes. Remove from the heat and set aside to cool. In a large bowl, add the shrimp, arugula, oil, lime juice, salt, and black pepper, and gently toss to coat. Serve immediately.

Shrimp, Apple & Carrot Salad

8 Servings

Preparation time: 18 minutes

Ingredients:

- 2 tbsps Dijon mustard
- 2 garlic clove, minced
- Freshly ground black pepper, to taste
- 6 cups apples, cored and sliced thinly
- 1 cup fresh mint leaves, chopped
- 0.5 cup olive oil
- 2 tbsps unsweetened applesauce
- Pinch of salt
- 4 tbsps fresh cilantro, chopped
- 24 medium shrimp
- 6 cups carrot, peeled and julienned
- 4 tbsps organic apple cider vinegar

Directions:

- In a large pan of boiling water, add shrimp and cook for about 3 minutes.
- Drain the shrimp well and set aside to cool.
- After cooling, peel and devein the shrimps.
- In a large bowl, add cooked shrimp and remaining all ingredients except cilantro and gently stir to combine.

- Cover and refrigerate to chill for about 1 hour.
- Top with cilantro and serve.

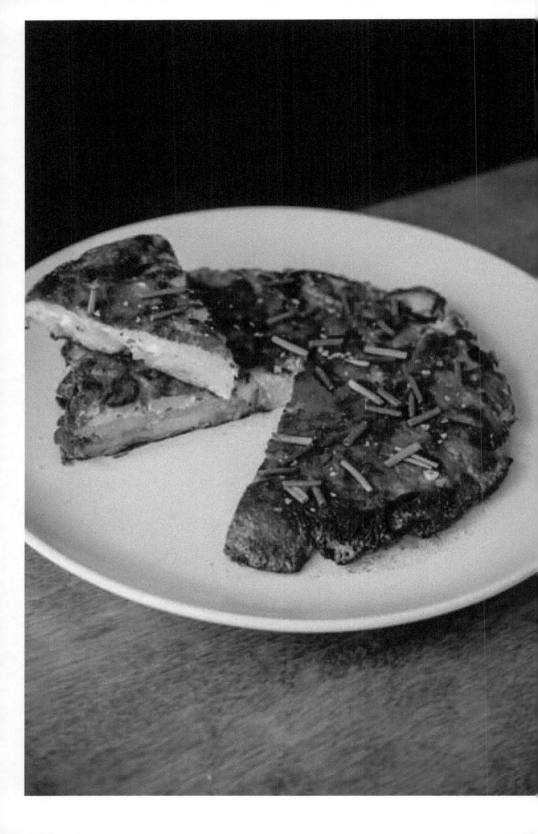

4 Servings

Preparation time: 20 minutes

Ingredients:

- 1 yellow onion, chopped
- 4 cups of water
- 1 teaspoon ground coriander
- 2 tablespoons fresh dill, chopped
- 1 teaspoon ground black pepper
- 1 tablespoon avocado oil
- 1 pound cod, skinless, boneless, and cut into medium chunks

Directions:

- Heat up a pot with the oil over medium-high heat, add onion, stir and cook for 4 minutes.
- Add all remaining ingredients and cook the soup for 20 minutes over medium heat.

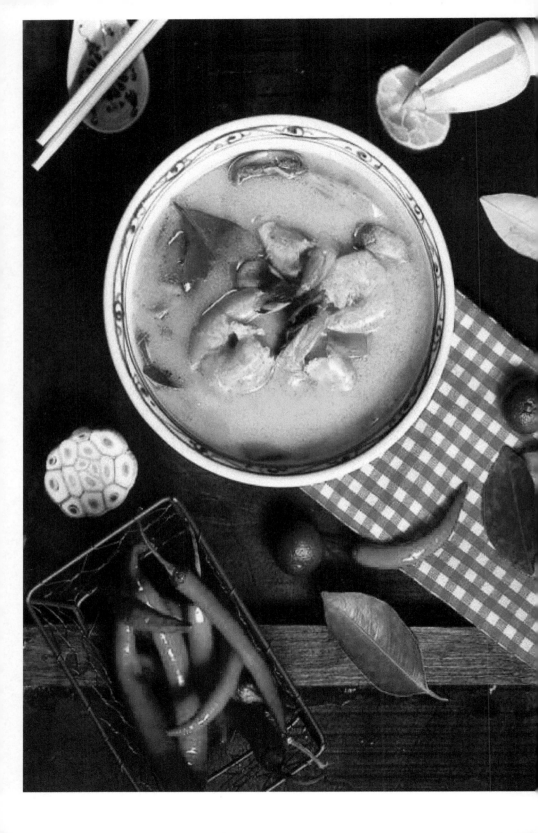

4 Servings

Preparation time: 25 minutes

Ingredients:

- 4 cups of water
- 1 pound trout fillets, boneless, skinless, and cubed
- 1 tablespoon sweet paprika
- 1 tablespoon olive oil
- 1 bell pepper, chopped
- 2 oz celery stalk, chopped

Directions:

- Heat up a pot with the oil over medium-high heat; add the celery stalk, stir and sauté for 5 minutes.
- Add the fish and all remaining ingredients and simmer the soup over medium heat for 20 minutes.

6 Servings

Preparation time: 50 minutes

Ingredients:

- 2 pounds chicken breast, skinless and boneless and cubed
- 2 red bell peppers, chopped
- 1 tablespoon olive oil
- 2 cups quinoa, already cooked
- ¼ cupcilantro, chopped
- 2 tablespoons lemon juice
- ½ teaspoon ground black pepper
- 4 cups of water
- 1 cuplow-fat milk

Directions:

- Heat up a pot with the oil over medium-high heat, add chicken and cook it for 5 minutes on each side.
- Add all remaining ingredients except quinoa and cook the soup for 40 minutes.
- Then add quinoa, stir it well and cook for 15 minutes more.

4 Servings

Preparation time: 25 minutes

Ingredients:

- 2 big eggplants, roughly cubed
- 4 cups of water
- 2 tablespoons tomato paste
- 1 tablespoon olive oil
- 2 tablespoons parsley, chopped
- 1 teaspoon ground turmeric

Directions:

- Heat up a pot with the oil over medium heat, add eggplants and sauté them for 5 minutes.
- Add all remaining ingredients and cook the soup for 25 minutes more.

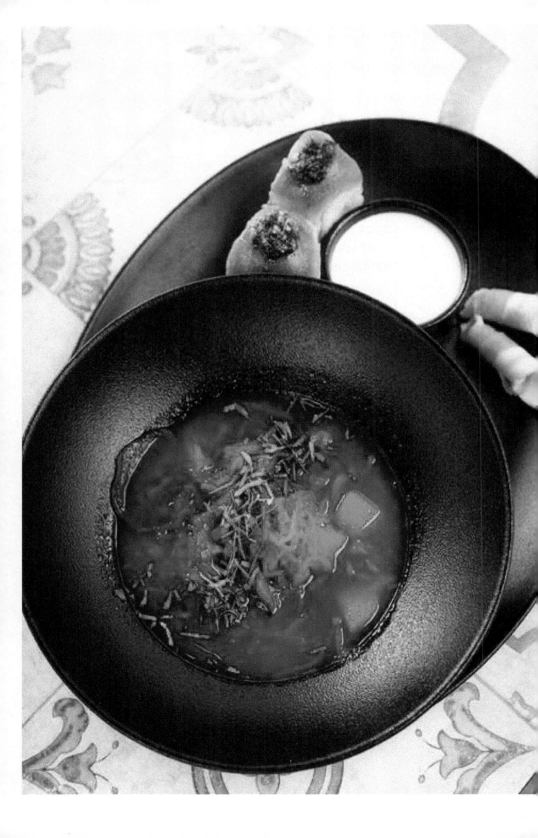